I0414193

NCD
Blue Bran Muffins

40% carbs 30% fat 30% protein and 500 calories

Number Crunch Diet Publications

ABC Water and the Number Crunch Diet
12 Changes A Year – Reality-Show Recipes

Other Publications

ABC Water and the Number Crunch Diet
a step by step solution to alkaline deficiency and
with a New and Unique approach to weight control

JPM Oral Hygiene Protocol
stop using toxic drugstore mouthwash, discover how to reduce
your gum pocket depth from 3-4-3 to 1-2-1 mm when they probe

NCD Flaxseed Shake Recipe
the Number Crunch Diet method for getting omega 3s
and with three variations so you'll never get bored

Nontoxic Teeth Whitening and Dental Hygiene System
"Spare me the chemicals, I've switched to FOOD GRADE to
whiten, gargle and brush."

The 5 Points of Posture
the missing link to fat loss, overall wellness, and
to becoming Respected, Adored, and Wealthy

12 Changes A Year – Volume 1
the recipe book to the Number Crunch Diet
When you take control of the numbers
you take control of your weight.

12 Changes A Year – Volume 2
the recipe book to the Number Crunch Diet
Begin today and forever be in control of the numbers you're eating.

12 Changes A Year – Volume 3
the recipe book to the Number Crunch Diet
You have to crunch the numbers to see what you're really eating.

Reality-Show RECIPES
12 Changes A Year – Vol. 1, 2, & 3
for the person who likes it real

Vision Is Possible
Improve your vision and get a facelift for free!
an original vision program targeting your Eye Lids

RAW MILK
the legal "Anabolic Steroid" for
common-sense Californians

GOOD Bacteria – Your Other Bodypart
looking deeper into your body's 2nd brain

NCD Lactose Intolerance Protocol
the Number Crunch Diet method to wean
yourself back on to milk

September 23, 2015 – The Rapture
Even if this date is wrong, you'll be ready for the next one.
What group are you in?

NCD Orange Shake
mmm! mmm! mmm!
The Number Crunch Diet uses real foods for flavor.

CONTENTS

To scroll through all 50 recipes, please visit

http://www.CreateSpace.com/6415380

Edits & Format

You will notice oddities in punctuation, spelling, syntax, and perhaps even semantics, within this book. Feel free to let me know, but some of it is done for brevity or to shift emphasis. I use capitals where I see fit, to grab your attention and make it stand out, and I also remove capitals when I don't think they are deserving of them, or to remove emphasis after first usage, i.e., Pyrex becomes pyrex. And french bread, brussels sprouts, and english cucumbers, are spelled lowercase, as we are not going to "link" a European vacation to our food and eating.

Secondly, I will unhyphenate to create rhythm. Grammatically, two or more words that function as an adjective before a noun are supposed to be hyphenated. That's fine. A million-dollar smile, is the adjective "million-dollar" describing the smile. However, this can get redundant after a while, 1&2 3, 1&2 3, 1&2 3. The noun gets all the attention. But what if you want the adjectives to have the emphasis? After all, the adjectives are the descriptive words. So, I will drop the hyphens to allow the adjectives equal emphasis, and to change the pace of the sentence a bit. So if there are no hyphens, read it slower and evenly, one two three four five six seven. A "step-by-step solution" sounds a bit skippy and simplistic, whereas, a "step by step solution" is said slower and sounds more methodical. Hyphenating two words, or joining two words as a compound word, reduces their individual meanings.

With regard to fastfood, healthfood, and seasalt, it's time for these words to evolve into compound words, so the trend starts here.

There are also some fragmented sentences, subject-verb disagreements, and singular/plural violations. When "correcting" certain of these sentences, they lost their emphasis and punch, so I kept them as is.

In the past I've been guilty of judging other author's sentences, only to reread it with the commas, pauses, and then it made perfect sense. So, if there's a comma, then pause, as you may not get to pause later in the sentence. If there's no comma, then don't pause and read it all as one.

I pose questions, but without question marks. Some are rhetorical, but some are to make you Ponder. Great word. Ponder. If you see a question mark at the end, then it requires an answer. If there's no question mark, then you can just say, yeah, no, or hm.

As I read comments made on the internet, I have come to the acceptance that an incomplete sentence or a prepositional phrase can actually stand alone as a sentence. For example, the comment, "Yes. In so many ways." A period instead of a comma, allows for a longer pause between the two, and so this is more accurately how someone might speak it. So a period can be used as a long pause, instead of "Yes, in so many ways."

The spelling of HomeGoods, PubMed, and others, has become common. You can now join two words and keep the capital.

Written English continues to change, people using it, customize the language to reflect exactly how they would speak it. It's a bit like ballroom dancing, the person leading gets to decide the movements and the pace, and each partner you dance with will use different movements and different paces. That said, I hope you enjoy this dance…

God Bless.

Steven Barry

You have to crunch the numbers to see what you're really eating.

Begin today and forever be in control of the numbers you're eating.

When you take control of the numbers, you take control of your weight.

Number Crunch Diet Publications – always profanity free

CHAPTER 1

Introduction

Woohoo!

Welcome to the Number Crunch Diet – Complete Nutrition, Maximum Freedom, Total Control. It's really the "All Your Dreams Come True Control Freak" diet. With a side of entertainment! But seriously, if you've tried the no-meat diet, or the no-carb diet, or the no-this diet no-that diet, then you are in for a treat. The NCD says: Eat it, and get it out of your system. And only the NCD says this.

In fact, after you've eaten everything you want, over and over again, you come to the place where – You Don't Want Anything Anymore. And you simply eat to supply your body with nutrition and energy. Of course there are some "rules", principles, and a brief summary will be provided in the next chapter.

Whereas the main book, *ABC Water and the Number Crunch Diet*, and the three cookbooks, *12 Changes A Year, Volumes 1, 2, and 3*, read like one giant 1000-page book, (so you can't really jump in anywhere and expect to fully understand it all, as it builds and flows from chapter to chapter), conversely, these NCD booklets are stand alone, you can read any one of the 50 booklets in any order.

Are you ready! I know you are! Let's pump this sucker out and get to it, but first we need "The Basics".

Chapter 2

The Basics

On the NCD, we count calories by counting pre-counted meals. Meaning that, you make a recipe, divide it up, and each serving, or meal, is 500 calories. The word "snack" means 250 calories.

Meal = 500
Snack = 250

You will only eat NCD meals and NCD snacks. So if you have 4 meals a day, you've had 4x500=2000 calories a day. If you have 5 meals a day, you've had 5x500=2500 calories a day. Six meals a day, 3000 calories. Seven meals, 3500 calories, and so on. For those of you that work physical jobs, you work on a fishing boat, or an oil rig, or you do yardwork 8-10 hours a day, then 4000 and 5000 and even 6000 calories a day is likely what your intake needs are. For these people, we have D-Meals, Double Meals, a double meal for breakfast, a meal and a shake for lunch, a double meal late-afternoon, and a double meal in the evening, 4x1000=4000.

If you're a woman working an office job, then your day might look like this:
Breakfast – 500
break – 250
Lunch – 500
break – 250
Dinner – 500

2000 calories a day, spread out throughout the day, 2-3-4 hours apart. There are lots of options for how you can consume your daily calories, and how to cut calories, and for that you will have to read the main books. But that gives you, The Basics.

Next, we will take a close look at the label of every food product we purchase, as that food is going into your body, and your body has to make new cells from that food, or detoxify any of the bad stuff that's in it. Preachers will say, the Bible is the "good news", but when it comes to your body, the "good news" is your liver. On the NCD we are allowed bad ingredients Rarely to Occasionally only. Not in moderation. The NCD says, "Moderation is too much." And, if you're a wine drinker, you need to cut that out. Drinking alcohol is a scam. It dehydrates your body and makes you age. Pomegranate juice contains just as much polyphenols and resveratrol as wine, as does simple grape juice. The NCD has a no alcohol rule. See the NCD Chicken Alfredo recipe for how to wean yourself off of red wine.

Young people, you are being scammed by the media and our culture into thinking that drinking alcohol and partying is fun. It's not. Do it, try it, and then move on. They are fooling you. You lose. The NCD is a health diet, so expect some lecturing. You will never fulfill your potential and purpose for being born if you waste your time drinking and partying on your days off. So, get busy. Set some goals. And focus in on them, like a laser beam. :)

Of all the people out there that read books, I would say 80% are women, so men, you've got some catching up to do.

And by books, I mean useful material, self-help, self-improvement. Christians spend time reading the Bible, and then call into a radio program crying because they've been diagnosed with cancer and are devastated and helpless. When someone says, "pray for me," hand them a self-help book and tell them to read their way out of their situation and trial. God has never failed me, He has always taken me through, BUT, I had to take action, I had to do it. He guides, you do.

Reading results in knowledge, then from there you can take Action.

Faith is not: God will come through. Faith is: God will guide your footsteps, and if you do it, you will come through. But in order to take action, you first need ample knowledge about your situation, otherwise, you are "destroyed", Hosea 4:6.

The NCD is a holistic diet, body mind soul spirit, whole body.

Although most of the recipes are 40 30 30, the NCD utilizes other macro percents as well, this is outlined in the main books. However, your day-in day-out macros should be 40 30 30. Everything you put in your mouth will be 40 30 30. Later, if you want to use different macros for different situation, then absolutely, go-for-it. But to start, just stick to 40 30 30. It's steady and stable, almost a-third a-third a-third, with a slight tip towards the carbs. If you want to argue or debate me on macro percents, read the main books first. I'm giving you the basics here.

So again, no bag of chips as a snack, everything you put in your mouth will be 40 30 30, and either 500 calories, or half, 250.

There aren't a lot of snack recipes on the NCD, so when you want a snack, just have half a meal. The NCD soups are great for cutting calories. They are 250 calories, but they fill you up like a 500 calorie meal. So, have the NCD French Onion soup for breakfast, and cut your breakfast calories from 500 to 250. But regular soups won't do it, as they are not 40 30 30.

The macro ratios are the key.

Once you begin to eat only pre-counted meals and snacks, then you can easily track your daily calories, as previously discussed. And once you know your calorie requirement, then you have control.

To do this, you must make a goal that you will continue to build your recipe repertoire until 100% of your eating comes from homemade meals you prepare yourself. No meals of unknown calories. This needs to be your goal. In the beginning, if you are in a pinch, you can, for example, walk over to the vending machine at work and have a regular-sized snickers bar, about 280 calories, just say 250. So this is your midmorning snack. But your goal is to prepare meals, all 40 30 30 and 500, and then bring meals and half-meals (snacks) to work so that 100% of your eating is 40 30 30.

Again, the reasons and the options are explained in the main books.

Trust me, I've been working on this diet for 15 years, perfecting the principles, expanding the options, and weeding out bad for good.

The Number Crunch Diet is not a get-thin-quick scheme. The recipe books are titled 12 Changes A Year on purpose, so, once a month, start a new recipe, make it again, then, next month repeat the cycle. At the end of one year, you should have 12 recipes in your repertoire. At the end of two years, 24 recipes, and at the end of three years, 36 recipes. Bingo! You're there. Goal: achieved. You will be eating 100% of your food from homemade meals you prepare yourself, from well-chosen grocery store items.

Hence, Complete Nutrition – Maximum Freedom – Total Control.

There's more that needs to be said, but let's just jump in and start, you will figure out the rest as you go. The best way to learn is to just, jump in. Dog paddle until you can swim! Let's go!

Chapter 3

The Items

The items you select to eat are important, as is how you cook them. You are what you eat, was true yesterday, is true today, and will still be true tomorrow.

If you eat animal muscle (meat), with the preservative sodium nitrite, you end up with nitrosamides (cancer).

If you cook that animal muscle (meat) at high temperatures and char it, burn it, until it's got black marks, you create polycyclic aromatic hydrocarbons (plastics).

Throw in a side of french fries deep fried in oil at 425°F, and you're eating acrylamides (cancer).

And if you chase that charred burger patty or flame-broiled chicken with a diet soft drink (aspartame), you create heterocyclic amines.

So the NCD takes a close look at what we are eating, we read the entire label:
1. the ingredients list
2. the nutrition facts numbers
3. the label bragging ("our product is …")

The fastest way to cut out all of those cancer-causing compounds listed above, is to eat your food RAW, the NCD is about 80% raw.

This recipe requires 9 different items, it makes 12 meals, x4=48.
1. flour
2. bran
3. hemp
4. blueberries x4
5. molasses
6. milk

7. whipped butter x4

8. chicken
9. FSP coating

As stated in the main books, if you live in California, well lucky you, as you will recognize these supermarkets, but clearly, I cannot shop for items in every city in the world and tell you where to go. You will have to search for the same or similar items in your area.

1. King Arthur Flour, 100% Whole Wheat, 5 lbs 2.27Kg, $4.79 at Smart & Final. Ingredients: 100% hard red whole wheat flour.

Choose a flour with one ingredient, and no iron or B vitamins added, as that indicates it's refined. We will be using 330g of this flour for 12 meals, so for 48 meals, we need a total of 330gx4=1320g, or a bit more than half the bag.

The nutrition facts for this item (in the United States) looks like this:

1/4 cup 30 grams
Servings about 76
Calories per serving = 100
Calories of Fat = 5
Fat = 0.5g
Saturated Fat = 0g
Trans Fat = 0g
Cholesterol = 0mg (milligrams)
Sodium = 0mg

Carbohydrate = 20g
Fiber = 4g
Sugar = 0g
Protein = 4g

People in Canada, Australia, the UK and elsewhere, your label may or may not have all these listed, or it may say Kcal, Kilo calories. Don't worry, just follow along. I like the U.S. nutrition facts label the best, however, they are planning on changing it and the proposed new label is…not that great.

So as you can see, the label has two units of measure, calories and grams. On the NCD we convert grams into calories, see below:

Fat grams to calories = times by 9
Carb grams to calories = times by 4
Protein grams to calories = times by 4

So, 9 4 4.

Also, the nutrition facts list the fat, then the carbs, then the protein. However, when we refer to the macro percents, the order is carbs fat protein.

40 30 30 is Carbs Fat Protein, so just be aware that the label has the Fat first.

None of the NCD recipes contain trans fat, so you won't see that number again. And saturated fat and cholesterol are both within normal limits on the NCD, so you won't see those again either.

So, I'm going to recrunch the label into calories, and write it all on one line. E=100 F=5 Na=0 CHO=80 f=16 s=0 Prot=16 T=101.

E = Energy, in calories
F = Fat, in calories
Na = sodium, in milligrams
CHO = Carbs, in calories

f = fiber, in calories
s = sugar, in calories
Prot = Protein, in calories
T = the total calories (Fat + Carbs + Protein)
T-f = T (total calories, fat+carbs+prot) minus the fiber

I go over this in full detail in the main books, but for this recipe, you don't really need to master all the calculations and numbers, but you should try to familiarize yourself with them. It's just one of the things in life a person should know and be familiar with.

Before we move on, I want you to notice that the calories are given at the top (100), but you can calculate it yourself by adding together the three items that have calories, Fat Carbs Protein (101).

This is how we double-check the accuracy of the label, E and T should match, or be close.

T-f. T is the total calories (fat+carbs+prot), and f is the fiber calories. Fiber comes in two forms, soluble and insoluble. The insoluble fiber doesn't enter your body, it stays within the colon, thereby, adding bulk to your stool. The soluble fiber gets absorbed into your body, but it creates a gel gelatin-like matrix that slows down the release of sugar into the bloodstream.

On the NCD, we subtract the fiber calories from our numbers.

So T-f is total calories minus the fiber, in this case, 101-16=85.

We also subtract the fiber from the carbs number, in this case, 80-16=64, and we call this number nCHO, net carbohydrates.

Lastly, we look at the macro percents of each food item. 40 30 30 is the macro percent of the meal, but each food item has its own percents.

To calculate the percent of something, you take the portion and divide it by the whole, times 100. With this food item, we have

5/101x100=5% fat, 80/101x100=79% carbs, and 16/101x100=16% protein, 79 5 16.

We have 3 things that make up the whole. Fats Carbs Protein

And they add up to the total calories, E, Energy. (and T)

I'll stop there, as I don't want to go too deep. It is all covered in progressive steps, with repetition, so that you will be a number crunch expert at the end. Your kids will be amazed by you!

And again, I've simplified the statements and rounded off the numbers. This is a booklet, not a book.

Now let's look at the third and final part of our food item, the label bragging. If you shop at the healthfood store, you will immediately notice that the food items have a lot of label bragging, and often true and important scientific facts. Many companies are catching on that in order to be competitive, they have to brag about their product and tell you what's good in it and why you should buy theirs over other brands. Some bragging is fake, for example, ketchup or Worcestershire sauce saying "fat free" on the label. Everyone knows that. Plus good fats are good for you, so a diet that is "fat free" is not a healthy diet. And we all know this now.

Fat Free is one of the many mainstream media scams. In the 1990s, doctors put their overweight patients on fat-free diets, which can only mean one thing – you eat more carbs. One woman I worked with said when she went back to her doctor a month later, she had gained 5 pounds.

Fat Free also means dry skin, as your cell membranes are dry.

Saturated fat is actually a great fat for soft hair and soft skin.™

And saturated fat is a natural fat, it's unprocessed. All vegetable oils, including olive oil, are processed. Read the front cover of *12 Changes A Year* (volume two).

On the NCD we eat 30% fat, and a balance of plant & animal fats.

Keep in mind that you cannot make two kinds of fat; omega-3 flax, and fish fat DHA EPA. I encourage you to read up on this fully.

Our WW flour says, "never bleached, never bromated, no preservatives", and "wheat is a Non-GMO product". Good.

When it comes to grains, the NCD likes to check the percent fiber.

NCD Whole Grain Rule, the percent fiber has to be double digit.™

With this flour, we have 16/101x100=16%, double-digit fiber percent, so it's a true whole grain.

Refined grains often have B vitamins and iron added, so if you see thiamine mononitrate et cetera in the ingredients, it's a refined grain. You will have refined grains on the NCD sometimes, and we call them "fun carbs".

330g of flour divide by 12 is, 27.5g E=92 F=5 CHO=73 f=15 s=0 Prot=15, rounded. Note, for our final numbers, we will add all of our ingredients together and divide by 12 at the end, so it will be more accurate, (but it's also nice to see the per meal amount).

2.   Wheat Bran, Bob's Red Mill brand, 20oz 567g, Lassen's Healthfoods Store, buy one, $2.49. Ingredient: wheat bran.

1/4 cup 15g
Serving per container 37
E=50cal
F=5cal
total Fat = 0.5g (x9 = 4.5cal) (close to 5)
Na=0mg
CHO=10g (x4 = 40cal)
f=2g (x4=8cal)
s=0g
Prot=2g (x4=8cal)

T=5+40+8=53cal (close to E=50 above)

Notice that the fat is given in calories (5), and in grams (0.5g). On the NCD, we use the Fat Cals number (5cal), and not the grams number, (0.5gx9cal=4.5cal).

And then our percents are, 5/53x100=9% fat, 40/53x100=76% carbs, 8/53x100=15% protein, 76 9 15.

Is this a true whole grain? Let's crunch it: 24/53x100=45% fiber.

Label bragging says, "unprocessed" and "an excellent source of fiber". Yeah, it's about half fiber, plus some naturally-occurring vitamins and minerals. It also says, "free of preservatives and chemical additives". We like that, ("free of chemical additives").

The "best-by" date was 24 months from the date I bought it, so it's fresh. We are going to use one-fourth of the bag for 12 meals, so, the entire 20oz bag for 48 meals, with none left over.

Typically, I will make 12 meals each week, and have two of these meals a day, say, 07:00 and 11:00. Since I need a minimum of 35 meals a week, these 12 meals are about a third of what I need for the week. And trust me, you won't get bored having this every week for the next four weeks. It's a party meal. Mmmm!

The front label says 20oz 567g, and when I weighed it, it was 590g, and the empty bag was 14g, so 590-14=576g. You get 576-567=9 extra grams. So, weigh your bag of bran, subtract 14g for the bag, and divide by 4, and that's how much you will use per batch of 12. In this case, 576÷4=144g, so use 144 grams per batch of 12.

For our numbers, we will use their stated 567÷4=142g divide by 12 meals equals 12g E=39 F=4 CHO=32 f=19 Prot=6.

If you buy two of the 10oz 283g bags, the empty bag is 7g, so place both bags on the scale, subtract 14g, and that's how much bran you really have. Then use 1/4th, (about 142-144 grams per 12 meals).

3.   Hemp Protein Powder, Bob's Red Mill brand, 16oz 454g, Lassen's, buy one, $13.99. Ingredient: hemp protein powder.

The nutrition facts say:
2 Tbsp 14g
Servings about 32
E=50cal
F=15cal
total Fat=1.5g (x9=13.5cal) (but we will use 15 above)
Omega-3=216mg
Na=0mg
CHO=4g (x4=16cal)
f=3 (x4=12cal)
s=1g (x4=4cal)
Prot=6g (x4=24cal)
T=15+16+24=55cal
29 27 44 (29% carbs, 27% fat, 44% protein)

Hemp powder is 44% protein. Good. It is also #3 for omega-3 fatty-acid content, Flax, Chia, Hemp. See the NCD Orange Chicken recipe in *12 Changes A Year (Vol. 1)* for more on this. Suffice it to say, fresh hemp powder is a superfood; high in protein, essential omega-3, plus minerals.

When I opened the bag, it was a beautiful hunter green color, fluffy and fresh, with a strong wonderful hemp smell. Wow.

The next time I made this recipe, something told me to check the hemp powder in the vitamins section, and so I purchased the Nutiva brand in the 16oz 454g container for $13.49 on sale, regularly $20.89. However, I didn't save any money because you have to pay tax on products purchased in the vitamin department, so it was $1.01 more with tax, $14.50.

Sometimes God has me do something, and in the moment, I don't know why, but later I come to understand. So the bottom line is: don't buy this in the vitamin section because it's a bit dry looking. People are putting this into shakes, so the company dries the hemp powder in order to make it more neutral smelling. As a result, it looks fine, but not beautiful. Instead of being a rich dark green, it's a dull-ish gray green, and not nearly as much of the amazing smell.

So, don't buy the one in the vitamin section, buy the one in the grocery aisle, in the same place as the wheat bran.

Regular supermarkets likely don't carry it, so if you don't have a healthfood store, you can buy Bob's brand online at Amazon.com.

Underneath the nutrition facts, it lists some mineral data. The Nutriva brand says that a 3 Tbsp 30g serving has 40% the RDA for iron, 25% the RDA for zinc, and 60% the RDA for magnesium.

The Recommended Daily Allowance for magnesium is 400mg, so 3T 30g has 240mg of magnesium. So when you think hemp, think minerals, #3 for omega-3, and protein. Plus rich green color.

We are using 4oz 113g per 12 meals, and this is why we are making this recipe 4 weeks in a row, so that when we are done, we have no hemp remaining, (4oz x4=16oz or 113.5gx4=454g).

Nutriva also says:
Non-GMO
Non-BPA container (bisphenol-A, "bad" plastic that leaches)
Organic
Made without hexane (a solvent used to extract certain cooking oils used in the deep fryers at fastfood outlets to cook french fries).

Bob's brand doesn't say organic, but I am pretty sure it's all coming from the same place in Canada, and they don't use pesticides there, (from what I was told by a cherry farmer in British Columbia).

Just remember that certification costs money, and some good companies, like Bob's Red Mill, are big on quality and honesty, so if the company is honest and good, then you can be confident that their products are not tainted and poisonous. So pay attention to the company, and $upport those that are good and honest.

Lastly, as you continue on your journey, you will come to discover that protein is not everywhere. Fats and carbs are everywhere, but protein is not everywhere. And, you will also discover as you read labels, that foods with a lot of protein cost more. Protein is "expensive". More expensive than fat and carbs. So when you see a product that has protein, just be aware that it will likely cost more. The bag of bran was $2.49, a lot less money than hemp.

For our meal, 4oz 113g divided by 12 meals is about 9.5g E=34 F=10 Omega-3=146mg CHO=11 f=8 s=3 Prot=16.

4. Blueberries, First Street brand, Smart & Final market, freezer section, 32oz 907g (a 2 lb bag), buy 4, use one per week, $7.99 x4=$31.96. In addition to protein being "expensive", anything that's good-for-you is also expensive. Ingredient: blueberries.

1 cup 140g
Servings about 6
E=70
F=5
Na=0
CHO=17g=68cal
f=4g=16cal
s=12g=48cal
Prot<1g=0 (the "<" sign looks like an L, for less than)
T=5+68+0=73

Of all the frozen blueberries available in my city, this brand is the best. They are big, 100% perfect, and delicious. We will use one bag per 12 meals, so each meal is about 76g E=38 F=3 Na=0 CHO=37 f=9 s=26 Prot=0, 93   7   0, 93% carbs, 7% fat (but probably no fat), and 0% protein. The fiber is 22% (16/73x100). So blueberries are another superfood, super high in antioxidant power, blue plant food, and 22% fiber, and low in calories, the 2-pound bag is 454 calories (using E), and T is close (907÷140x73= 473cal). With the fiber subtracted, T-f is only 369 calories per 2lb.

Keep 3 bags in the freezer, and thaw 1 bag overnight in the fridge.

Just briefly, if the nutrition facts are for 140 grams, and we want 76 grams, we have to divide 76 grams by 140 equals 0.54, and we multiply the nutrition facts by 0.54, 70x0.54=38, 5x0.54=3 68x0.54=37 et cetera. But again, we will add it all up at the end and divide by 12 at the end to get our final numbers.

Okay,
330g flour (2 ¾ cups)
5oz wheat bran (142g) (or 144g if they gave you extra)
4oz hemp (113g) (or 120g if they gave you extra)
32oz blueberries

As with the wheat bran, the Bob's hemp powder weighed more than 454g, it was 493g, and the bag is 10g, so you get 483g, or about 29 extra grams. Just turn on your scale, place the bag of hemp on the scale, toggle from ounces to grams, if your number says 490g, then subtract 10g for the bag, equals 480g, and divide by 4 = 120g, so just use 120g per batch instead of 113g.

You'll need a kitchen scale, I recommend the Taylor TE10C from Smart and Final for $55. It plugs into the wall outlet, so it will stay on until you shut it off. The battery-operated scales will shut off after 30 seconds and so you may lose your number while you prep.

5. Molasses, Blackstrap, Plantation brand, Lassen's, 31 fl oz, 915 mL, glass bottle, buy one, $7.79. Ingredient: unsulphured blackstrap molasses. 1T 21g E=42 F=0 Na=10 K=600 CHO=11g f=0 s=11g Prot=0g T=44, 100 0 0.

In the *NCD Flaxseed Shake Recipe*, I show the difference between this molasses, the organic molasses, and the regular store-bought molasses. Bottom line: this brand is the only one that came in glass, it had the highest mineral percents, and the lowest carbs, hence, it is the most robust and least refined, so buy this one. The regular supermarket brand is garbage, (90% less minerals).

The above book is probably one of the best books ever written, and every person should read it, but sadly, almost no one has.

K is potassium, primarily found in fruits and vegetables, and in this unrefined sugar product. Fruits and vegetables are also where we get bicarbonate. The nutrient no one talks about, except JPM.

Potassium is not usually listed on the nutrition facts, but because this molasses is high in potassium, they have listed it, and they brag on the label, "significant source of iron, calcium and potassium". All true. But not if you buy the common brand.

Potassium RDA = 3500mg, $600 \div 3500 \times 100 = 17\%$, and we are having 21g of this molasses per meal so we are getting 17% of our RDA of potassium per meal, plus 20% the RDA for calcium, and 20% the RDA for iron.

Potassium balances out the sodium in our diet, so pay some attention to getting potassium in your diet.

We will add 252g of this molasses to our batch, and so this bottle will be enough for all 4 batches, with about $1/5^{th}$ of the bottle left over that we will use in the NCD Flaxseed Shake.

6. 2% Milk, 16oz 488g, Berkeley Farms, or any other good brand, one quart is $1.69, use half for the recipe and have the remaining 16oz as a 40 30 30 snack (250cal). Since I drink a quart of milk a day, I buy a gallon of 2% milk, use 16oz 488g for the batch, and then I have 3 quarts and 16oz left over, so 3 meals (3x500) and 1 snack (1x250). Or you can buy a 16oz carton of 2% milk, 1 per week x4.

The nutrition facts say, 1cup 240mL (which weighs 244g), E=140 F=45 Na=150 K=460mg CHO=14gx4=56 f=0 s=13gx4=52 Prot=10gx4=40 T=141, 40 32 28. Almost 40 30 30.

Notice that one cup of milk has nearly a half a gram of potassium. 2% Milk is 3 Things: 40 30 30, minerals, hydration. Excellent.

5. Whipped Butter, Challenge brand, Smart & Final market, 8oz 227g, buy 4, $3.39x4=$13.56, use one per week   Ingredients:

pasteurized cream, (milk), salt.

Nutrition Facts:
1T (tablespoon) 9g
Servings per container 25
E=70cal
F=70cal
Na=58mg
CHO=0
Prot=0
T=70

Butter is 100% fat, 70÷70x100=100%. Regular butter that is not whipped is 100 calories per tablespoon and 14 grams. But because they have whipped it, it's lighter, a tablespoon is 5 grams lighter (9g) and 30% less calories (70 instead of 100). Restaurants like to use whipped butter because you can have more of it, and it tastes better whipped. If you can't find whipped butter, use the same number of grams of regular butter. The healthfood store used to sell organic whipped butter but they don't anymore, and many regular supermarkets don't carry it.

We are going to use 15 grams per meal, E=117 F=117 Na=97.

If you use regular unwhipped butter, 14g = 100cal, then use 15g.

They brag that it's from cows not treated with rBST growth hormone. Funny how nearly all the milk now is non-rBST. People don't want artificial growth hormones in their dairy products.

To soften it, remove it from the fridge 30 minutes before use. We want it soft and fluffy so we can spread it on both muffins, and if it's hard, it won't spread.

Okay, 330g flour, 142g wheat bran, 113g hemp, 907g blueberries, 252g molasses, 488g 2% milk, and 15g butter (whipped or nonwhipped). That's our muffins. Let's put it together in the next chapter. Then we'll add a side of chicken for protein.

Chapter 4

Muffin Prep

If you are new to baking, just think of it like this: add the dry ingredients to a bowl, add the wet ingredients to another bowl, mix the wet into the dry, and bake. Simple.

On the NCD, we weigh things instead of using measuring cups and measuring spoons, it's faster, less dishes to wash, and more accurate. So, place a large bowl on your scale, now turn it on, it will read zero. Add 330 grams of WW flour. Now press "tare" and the scale will read zero again. Now add 142g of wheat bran. Now press tare, it will read zero, now add 113g of hemp. Press tare, it will read zero, add 25g of baking soda (4t, measuring teaspoons). Press tare, it will read zero, add 6g salt (1t, measuring teaspoon).

All teaspoons are level, you swipe the back of a knife across the measuring spoon to level it. Also, 4t = 1Tbsp+1t.

Mix this bowl of dry thoroughly with a whisk. Set aside.

Add the two pounds of thawed blueberries to a wave blender, (in the photo you can see the pitcher has a groove, so the contents shoot up the side and down onto the blade). Place the pitcher on the scale, press tare, add 252g of molasses. Then press tare to zero the scale, and add 488g of 2% milk. Blend until smooth (60sec).

Pour the pitcher of wet into the bowl of dry and mix well.

At this point, your batter looks black because of the blueberries, but when the muffins are cooked, they will look chocolate brown.

Your bowl of raw muffin batter should be 80.4 ounces or 2281g, divide by 12 equals 190g per meal, divided by 2 equals 95g per muffin.

So, place the glass pyrex bowl on the scale, use a soupspoon to add 95g of batter (two spoonfuls), repeat 23 more times.

The photo on the front cover shows the muffins in the blue lid bowls, and the chicken in the red lid bowls. Both bowls are 1cup 236mL in size. The red-lid bowls are Pyrex brand, and the blue-lid bowls are Anchor brand. Either brand is fine for baking in.

Okay, you have 24 small glass bowls with 95 grams of batter in each bowl, or plus/minus a gram or two, no biggie.

I bake these in my large Hamilton Beach toaster oven. It has 4 rack positions, and I place 8 bowls on each of the 3 bottom racks, so, rack one (top position) is empty, then rack two has 8 bowls, then rack three has 8 bowls, and rack four (the bottom position) has 8 bowls, 8+8+8=24 bowls.

Close the oven door, set it to "Bake" and 350°F, and start a timer.

At 20:00 (20 minutes), remove the bottom rack and place it on top of the oven, then move the third rack to the bottom, and move the second rack to the third position, and then slide the bottom rack into position two.

At 40:00, rotate the racks again, 4 to 2, 3 to 4, and 2 to 3.

At 60:00, turn off the oven and open the door.

Set your time again. At 60:00, remove all the bowls to the counter.

Set your timer again. At 60:00, cover with the lids and refrigerate.

So,
60:00 in the oven at 350
60:00 in the oven with it turned off and the door open
60:00 on the counter
Cover and Refrigerate

When you open the oven door, the muffins fall, making them dense. Then when you cover them with the lids and refrigerate, you lock in the moisture. Dense and Moist, mmmmmmm!

You can have a meal now, while they are still warm, and then the remaining 11 meals the muffins will be refrigerator temperature.

Use a plastic knife to circle around the bowl twice, turn the bowl upside down, and it will fall out in one piece. Place two muffins on a plate, place the plate on the scale, press tare or on, it will read zero, now add 15 grams of butter, about half on each muffin.

Whichever way you decide to bake them, take notes so that you can perfect the procedure. If you do it exactly as above, all 24 muffins will be dense and moist and they will fall out of the bowl in one piece after you circle around the edge of the muffin 360 degrees 2x.

Use a strong plastic dinner knife, as you don't want to scratch the glass bowl by using a metal knife. You can use a metal dinner knife, but flip it around and use the backside to circle the bowl.

When you are filling the bowls with the 95g of batter, tap or hit the side of the bowl with the heel of your hand to level the batter if it's not flat. They are nicer if they are the shape of hockey pucks, and not like tennis balls (rounded on top, like store-bought muffins).

So picture it: chocolate brown muffins, that are dense and heavy-ish, but super moist when you sink your teeth into them, and topped with almost a tablespoon of whipped butter on each one. Ah! La La land. You won't mind having two of these a day for the next month. But you need some protein to make this a meal, and to sustain you until your next meal 3-4 hours from now.

Chapter 5

FSP Chicken

I'll admit, that was a bit of work, but let's look at the benefits: WW flour with one ingredient, Wheat Bran with one ingredient, Hemp powder, a superfood, Blueberries, a superfood, Plantation brand Molasses, another superfood. This is ten-times better than any cereal you would have for breakfast, and now we are going to add some protein to make it a meal, because without the chicken, it's a dessert, and the numbers prove it, see below:

2 muffins
E=268
F=29
Na=35+ (plus a bit of sodium from the baking soda and salt)
K=677 (high potassium)
CHO=206
f=50cal=12.5 grams of fiber! (almost half the 30g RDA)
s=81
Prot=44
T=279
74 10 16 (74% carbs, 10% fat, 16% protein)

Now let's top them with 15g of whipped butter! Mmm!
E=385 F=146 CHO=206 Prot=44 T=396, 52 37 11.

Luckily, the hemp and the whole wheat flour are providing some protein, otherwise, this would be about 50 50 carbs and fat, dessert.

On the NCD, we get to eat desserts and carb-fat combinations, but we balance it with a portion of protein. This is key. It's nutrition.

NCD FSP Coating™
Flour Salt Pepper

Place a 16oz jar on the scale, press on or tare to zero it, now add flour until it says 180 grams. Next, add 17g of finely ground black pepper, and then 32g of Lawry's Seasoned Salt No MSG. Be sure to buy the seasoned salt that says "No MSG" on the front. Although it does contain "Natural Flavors" which is basically a code word for addictive chemicals.

So the healthier, less chemically-risky version of the FSP Skillet Chicken™ is to substitute sea salt for the Lawry's Seasoned Salt. I have switched to the sea salt version and it tastes almost the same. However the seasoned salt does make the chicken taste more like KFC (Kentucky Fried Chicken). Or, you can do 50/50, use 16g of sea salt and 16g of Lawry's seasoned salt.

For the measuring people, it's:
1 ¼ cups flour
2T finely ground black pepper (be sure it's finely ground)
2T salt (sea salt, or 50/50)
Cap & Shake

The salt and pepper have no calories, but we will count the flour. We will estimate that each serving gets sprinkled with 9g of flour, but that we lose about a third of it to the skillet, and so we are eating 6g of flour, E=20 F=1 Na=0 CHO=16 f=3 s=0 Prot=3. King Arthur has changed their nutrition facts slightly since 2014 when I published this recipe in the main books, and you will encounter this periodically here-and-there as you read labels for yourself.

And finally, Foster Farms Chicken Breasts, the 6-pack, $3.99/lb and we need 3 lbs trimmed, so buy 3.2lbs or 1.5Kg, $12.77. This is enough for our 12 meals, and then you will buy this again for weeks 2, 3, and 4. We are having 4oz raw 3.4oz cooked.

E=120
F=10
Na=75mg
CHO=0
Prot=26gx4=104
T=114

Be sure to check the sodium and that it's not 330mg or 470mg, as this indicates that the breasts are in 15% solution.

This foster-farms chicken says "up to 2% retained water" and no solution or ingredients, it's just boneless skinless chicken breasts.

Now cooked chicken and raw chicken do not weigh the same, so I have figured out the conversion by weighing it raw, cooking it in the skillet, then weighing it cooked.

NCD Skillet-Chicken Conversion™
Raw to Cooked = times 0.85
Cooked to Raw = divide by 0.85

So you lose about 15% after you cook it in a skillet, hence, 4oz x0.85 = 3.4oz cooked. But we also have the coating, so we will assume about 0.3oz for the coating, making our serving of FSP Skillet Chicken 3.7oz or 105g. E=140 F=11 Na=75+ CHO=16 f=3 Prot=107 T=134.

Remove the breasts from the package and use a scissors to trim off any visible fat, this foster-farms 6-pack has very little fat.

Next, if you bought the value-pack of chicken breasts for $2.49/lb, then you will need to flatten them between two cutting boards so that they are an even thickness, otherwise, the thin end of the breast cooks and gets overcooked, while the thick end of the breast is still raw in the middle. So flatten them to one-half inch thick.

The nice thing about the foster-farms 6-pack is that they have minimal fat to trim off and they are fairly flat so you don't have to flatten them.

Place the chicken in the skillet and sprinkle with the FSP coating, turn them over and sprinkle again. Now add 1 cup of water. Cover and cook at 350°F for 6 minutes, setting your timer. At 6:00, remove the cover and turn the breasts over, cover and cook 6 more minutes. At 12:00, unplug the skillet, remove the cover, and slice the chicken into strips on a cutting board, then slice coming back in the opposite direction so that the chicken is in cubes (diced).

Place a small pyrex bowl on the scale, zero it, add diced FSP Chicken until it says 3.7oz or 105g. If you want extra zing, you can scoop more of the coating from the skillet into your bowl. Continue making servings of chicken until you have 12, for 12 meals, (2 muffins, 15g butter, 3.7oz FSP chicken).

The final numbers are:

E=525cal
F=157cal   29.6%
Na=fine
CHO=222cal   41.9%
f=53   10.0%
s=81cal   15.3%
Prot=151cal   28.5%
T=530
T-f=477

So we are right around 500 calories, 530, and if we subtract the fiber calories, then 477. The macros are 42 30 28, but the net carbohydrates are 222-53=169. The meal feels just right. We've got some sugar there to keep us going so no sleepy brain, but no sugar spiking either. It's really a masterpiece of numbers. You will have no leftovers after 48 meals, except the 4th container of butter will have about 176g remaining. Make the NCD Buttered Popcorn recipe or the NCD Corn on the Cob recipe (11 meals) to use it up.

Price per meal is $2.56. Enjoy…

Leave a Review

If you are going to leave a review, first ask yourself:

1. Did the recipe target 40 30 30 and 500 calories? Yes it did.
2. Does the photo accurately depict the meal? Yes is does.
3. Was full disclosure made before you purchased? Yes it was.
    "With a side of entertainment!"
(and if you're not a fan, just quietly move on, you don't need to spoil it for others and turn people away by being negative)

www.amazon.com   Search: NCD Blue Bran Muffins

Subscribe to my YouTube Channel
www.youtube.com   ABC Water and the Number Crunch Diet

abcwaterandthenumbercrunchdiet@mail.com
Privacy – your email address will not be used for anything other than by Jumper Publications and Media.
www.abcwaterandthenumbercrunchdiet.com

Some of you may have caught on that I'm using a different name. Actually, those are my names, just in a different order. Amazon allows authors to have up to three bio pages, but they have to be different names, so I am able to double my exposure on their website by using a different name. It's similar to how Safeway, SuperValu, Vons, and Alberstons are all owned by Alberstons LLC.

Party On Dude

For those of you that want to read *ABC Water and the Number Crunch Diet*, but it's a bit expensive for you, if you send me a money order or PayPal payment I can mail you the book for 40% off the list price ($108) and free shipping.

Learn everything you need to know about alkalinity and acid-base.

NUMBER CRUNCH DIET

01	Rueben Sandwich
02	Soyaki Chicken
03	Blue Bran Muffins
04	Beef Stroganoff
05a	Corn on the Cob
05b	Cola Milkshake
06a	Beef Jerky Cookies
06b	Peanut Butter Chocolate
07a	Steak Baked Beans
07b	Raw-Egg Eggnog
08	Chicken Caesar Salad
09a	Beef & Rice
09b	Orange Juice Milk – ADM
09c	Melted Cheddar – ADM
10	Chicken Potato Salad
11a	Beef Dip
11b	2% Milk Perfected
12	check back later
13	to follow
14	pending
15	to be published soon
16	not available yet
17	coming soon
18	not yet available
19	to be released in the fall
20	oops, error 404
21	please try again
22	it's been a busy week (month)(year!)
23	I'm workin' on it
24	coming to a theater near you
25	check again later

NUMBER CRUNCH DIET

26	pending
27	please check again later
28	system maintenance
29	check back later
30	later dude
31	refresh
32	not responding
33	crash dump
34	reboot
35	please wait
36	please be patient
37	loading…
38	page not available
39	check back later
40	please try again later
41	laters
42	partial
43	in process
44	processing
45	please check back
46	future release date pending
47	not yet available
48	my guess is
49	you will
50	Check Back Later ;)

Build a NCD Recipe Repertoire

Body –> Mind –> Soul => Spirit

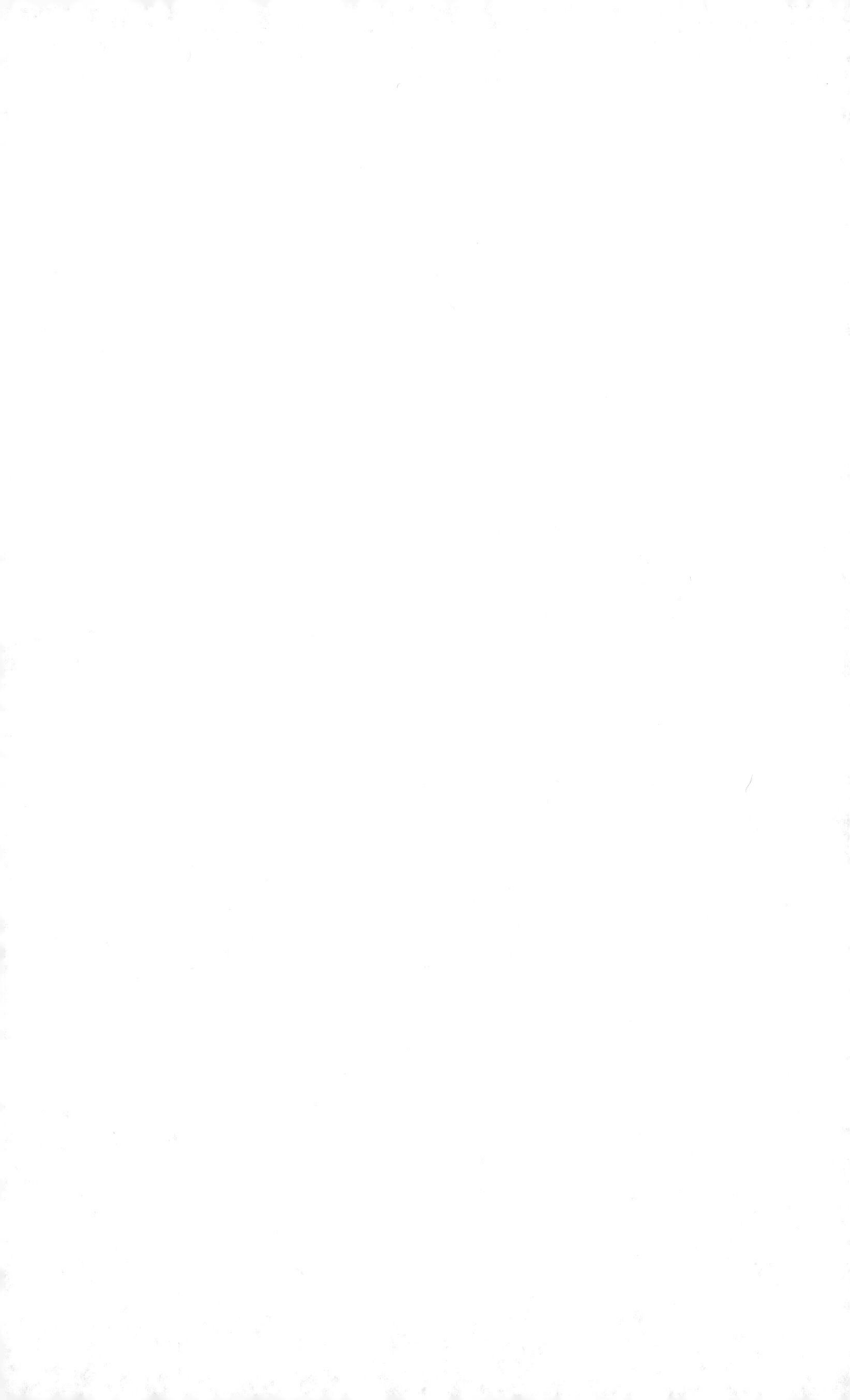